Chinese Herbal Remedies

Chinese Remedies to Treat the Most Common Ailments

Summary

- This book is intended to educate and motivate. With twenty five easy herbal recipes to cure common ailments that weaken the body, this book is to-the-point and complete.

- You don't have to read pages and pages of unwanted information; just skip through the table of contents for the ailment you are searching the cure for and the book will jot down the steps you need to follow in few easy steps.

- In order to facilitate readers, the book is written in easy, understandable English that facilitates its use further.

- Mostly, the recipes you will find in this book are soups and teas, so you done have to spend hours in the preparation of one recipe; what you will need to do is find the ingredient (the ingredients are also simple.

- In this book we have tried to incorporate as many easily and readily available ingredients as possible) and boil them in water in the prescribed manner. Ingredients like ginger and rice and turnips have been used that will not only cure the illness but it will also add taste.

- Special attention has been given to include recipes that are not only curing but also good to taste; therefore, you will find that brown sugar and honey has been widely used in the recipes to add sweetness and taste.

- Chinese herbal remedies have been used for centuries to cure and revitalize the human body, so why should you not give it a try and enjoy the health benefits that it has to bring. Because the ingredients are all herbal, you do not even have to worry about the side effects of the medicine.

- Knowledge acquired by the Chinese through the centuries has been conglomerated to device recipes that will cure ailments like diabetes for good, an ailment for which even modern doctors have no permanent solution for.

Contents

Introduction

Chinese herb-ology, the theory of traditional Chinese herbal therapies provides treatments from different ailments for centuries. The first recognized herbalist in Chinese herbology is Shénnóng and it dates back to 2800 BC.

Herbs used in treatment of ailments through Chinese remedies include mushrooms, cinnamons and ginger. Chinese medicines are 100% herbal and have been used to treat diverse ailments of acne, hair loss, asthma, cramps, flu and indigestion.

You will notice that most of the ingredients can easily be found in the market, you will not have to make any special effort with regards the attainment of the ingredients. Alternately, you can find the ingredients in health food or vitamin stores, online or the at the Chinese medical practitioners office.

For centuries, Chinese Herbal medicines have been used to treat patients with various illness, like you will read through in the book. The Chinese medications can be made easily by decocting ingredients in water; therefore, they do not usually require extensive effort. In this book, we will not only know how you will be able to make the medicine, you will also be guided regarding the recommended usage of the medicine.

Chinese medicine has been used for centuries to cure illnesses, and not the secret to those recipes is in your hands.

Acne

Caused by excessive oil production by the skin, acne is a common ailment especially among individuals reaching their puberty. Acne is characterized by red skin protrusions on the face with a burning sensation.

Chinese Remedy:

The Chinese remedy entails cooling the blood and clearing away pathogenic heat from the body.

Ingredients

   15 grams of loquat leaf

   9 grams of Capejasmine fruit

   9 grams of Red peony root

   9 grams of Moutan bark

   9 grams of Forsythia frut

   9 grams of Coptis root

   9 grams of Prunella spike

   15 grams of dried rehmannia root

   15 grams of Scrophularia root

   9 grams of Mulberry bark

9 grams of Scutellaria root

9 grams of White chrysanthemum flower

Instructions

1. Combine all the ingredients
2. Decoct in water
3. Serve.

How to Consume

Oral consumption, 1 cup a day for three days

Common Cold

Cold, also known as nasopharyngitis, is a contagious, yet self-limited ailment caused by a number of viruses. Common symptoms of cold include coughing with a sore throat, runny nose and sneezing.

Chinese Remedy:

Ingredients:

> one tablespoon of honeyone fourth teaspoon cinnamon powder

Instructions:

1. Take the honey and warm it in a microwave for a few seconds.
2. Stir in the honey to the cinnamon powder.

How to consume:

Ideally, consume orally for three days consecutively for best results.

Anemia

Anemia is the decrease of red blood cells in the body. The red blood cells carry oxygen to the body. Due to the decrease of hemoglobin in the blood anemia in patients is characterized by fatigue, heart palpitations and pale skin as the body does not have enough oxygen to carry out routine tasks.

Chinese Remedy:

Ingredients:

40 grams of maltose syrup

12 grams of cinnamon stick

4 slices of ginger

4 red dates

24 grams of white peony honey

Instructions:

1. Take four cups of water and boil the herbs.
2. Reduce to one cup.
3. Add in the maltose and serve.

How to consume:

Use at least five times, one cup daily. Oral consumption.

Jaundice

Jaundice is characterized by yellowness and paleness of the skin caused by increased amounts of bilirubin. The bilirubin is a yellow substance in the hemoglobin that causes the discoloration of the skin, including the eyes.

Chinese Remedy:

Ingredients:

    40 grams of dried hyersium

    two eggs with shells

Instruction:

1. Boil the eggs and dried hyersium in four cups of water until it is reduced to about two cups.
2. When it reduces to half, take out the eggs from the shell and boil for another a few minutes while the water reduces to one cup.
3. Add some salt for taste.
4. Drink the tea and eat the eggs.

How to consume:

Drink one cup daily. It should be used every day for at least ten days.

Diarrhea

Diarrhea is characterized by watery bowel movements. It is very common and can affect all ages.

Chinese Remedy:

Ingredients:

> 30 grams of astragalus
>
> 9 grams of Atractylodes Rhizoma
>
> 9 grams Chinese Yam
>
> 9 grams of Indian bread

Instructions:

1. Boil the herbs in a small pot in five cups of water and continue boiling until the tea reduces to one cup.
2. Strain the tea and have one cup a day.

How to consume:

Consume one cup daily for at least three days.

Constipation

In constipation a person is unable to pass out normal bowel movement, resulting in buildup of toxins in the body. Such toxins, if the ailment is not treated timely can spread throughout the body and manifest into bigger problems of arthritis, rheumatism, and high blood pressure.

Chinese Remedy:

Ingredients:

> 30 grams of kelp
> brown sugar(for sweetening)
> 40 grams of mung bean

Instructions:

1. Soak the kelp in water until it becomes soft.
2. Boil the ingredients in a small pot in four cups of water. Keep boiling until the soup reduces to one cup.
3. Serve one cup daily with brown sugar.

How to consume:

Ideally, you should consume one cup daily for at least five days or until symptoms improve. Oral consumption.

Sore Skin

Caused by the heat of the sun, sore skin affects children and adults alike. The heat, heats up the blood and soreness of the skin is experienced.

Chinese Remedy:

Ingredients:

> 15 grams of mung beans,
> 30 grams of job's tears,
> 60 grams of pork that you have cut into small pieces
> 200 grams of loofah

Instruction:

1. Boil the ingredients in six cups of water, make sure the pork is washed and cleaned and cut into bite s
2. Reduce the soup to two cups.
3. Add some salt.
4. Serve.

How to consume:

Consume orally. Serve one cup daily until symptoms improve.

Dry Eyes

Characterized by dryness and redness of the eyes, the symptoms of this ailment may include itchiness of the eyes and discomfort in sleeping. Dryness of the eyes is a common and treatable ailment.

Chinese Remedy:

Instructions:

> 10 grams of goji berries,
>
> 10 grams of mulberry,
>
> 10 dates,
>
> 10 grams of Chinese yam and
>
> salt to taste(Preferably use rock salt)

Instructions:

1. First, soak all the herbs in water for around fifteen minutes.
2. Then boil them in five cups of water and reduce to one cup.

3. Add some salt and drink one cup daily after straining.

How to consume:

Consume orally; one cup daily until symptoms improve.

Depression

Depression is caused by the aggravation of the vital energies of the mind. Depression can be manifested in many ways.

Chinese Remedy:

Ingredients:

    12 grams of licorine

    40 grams of wheat

    10 red dates

    120 grams of lean pork, cut into small pieces

Instructions:

1. Boil all the ingredients in a pot with eight cups of water.
2. Reduce to soup of two cups.
3. Add some salt.
4. Serve.

How to consume:

Consume orally; no restriction on the amount of consumption. Ideally have one cup a day until symptoms have improved.

Palpitation

This is a condition of perceived abnormality of the heartbeat and awareness of contraction of heart muscles on the chest.

Chinese Remedy:

Ingredients:

    40 grams of dried lily bulbs

    2 boiled eggs

    40 grams of rehmanaia (processed)

Instructions:

1. Include and boil the ingredients in three cups of water.
2. Reduce to one cup.
3. Add some honey for sweetness.
4. Serve daily with boiled eggs.

How to consume:

Consume orally. Un-shell the eggs and have one cup daily with eggs. Continue until symptoms improve.

Dry Cough

Dry cough does not even cause discomfort, it is an underlying symptom for chronic lung disease and virus.

Chinese Remedy:

Ingredients:

    10 fresh green olives and

    640 grams of turnip

Instructions:

1. Prepare soup by boiling the ingredients in five cups of water until the water reduces to two cups.
2. Season with salt and pepper if you want and serve.

How to consume:

Consume orally. No restriction on the consumption. However, ideally have two cups in a day for at least ten days.

Fatigue/ Dizziness

Fatigue and dizziness can be caused by a variety of reasons, including low blood pressure and lack of energy due to malnutrition.

Chinese Remedy:

Ingredients:

>   500 grams of cooked red dates
>   500 grams of walnuts
>   250 grams of maltose
>   120 grams of honey

Instructions:

1.   Cut dates and walnuts into small pieces.
2.   Mix in the dates and add in the honey.
3.   Refrigerate and cut into small cubes.
4.   Eat regularly as a snack.

How to consume:

Consume orally as a snack. No restriction.

Fever

Fever is characterized by rise in body temperature. Symptoms for fever may include dizziness and weakness, including headache and body pain.

Chinese Remedy:

Ingredients:

    ten grams of burdock

    10 grams of mulberry leaf

    100 grams of honey

    100 grams of rice, uncooked

Instructions:

1. Cook in a pot with three cups of water. Reduce the water to one cup. Keep this herbal tea aside.
2. Prepare rice congee by boiling rice in water until the rice gets mushy. Add herbal tea and honey to the rice congee. Mix and serve.

How to consume:

Orally, once a day for at least three days.

Unclear Vision

Unclear vision can be caused by a several underlying problems including high cholesterol and high blood pressure. Symptoms include blurry vision and difficulty in reading.

Chinese Remedy:

Ingredients:

> two dried abalone
> 640 grams of lean pork, cut into small pieces
> 15 grams of gastrodia
> 4 pieces of ginger
> 12 grams of goji berries

Instructions:

1. Soak the ingredients overnight.
2. Boil all the ingredients in ten cups of water for three hours.
3. Add seasoning and serve.

How to consume:

Consume orally once everyday, until symptoms improve.

Low Blood Sugar

Hypoglycemia, commonly known as low blood sugar level is characterized by low glucose level and insulin reaction. Symptoms of low blood sugar ranges from blurry vision, rapid heartbeat and unexplained fatigue.

Chinese Remedy:

Ingredients:

> 180 grams of Chinese celery
> 240 grams of mustard green
> 120 grams of dried mussels

Instructions:

1. Wash and rinse the ingredients and cut them into small pieces.
2. Cook 8 cups of water and cook for one hour.
3. Serve.

How to consume:

Consume orally at least once every day for ten days.

Indigestion

Indigestion causes upsetting of the stomach when the metabolism of the body is unable to break down food in your body. Reasons for indigestion range from lack of sleep to stress.

Chinese Remedy:

Ingredients:

> 20 grams of Hawthorn fruit
>
> brown sugar for sweetness
>
> 8 grams of immature Chinese orange
>
> 12 grams of barley malt

Instructions:

1. Boil the ingredients in four cups of water and reduce it to one cup.
2. Strain and serve one cup daily.

How to consume:

Consume orally at least once every day for five days.

Insomnia

Insomnia is characterized by sleeplessness. Reasons for insomnia range from stress, imbalanced diet to indigestion.

Chinese Remedy:

Ingredients:

> 15 grams of dried lily bulb
>
> 15 grams of Biota Orientalis
>
> 15 grams of Rehmannia Radix
>
> 20 grams of Chinese Jujube
>
> 30 grams of Licorice
>
> 100 grams of wheat

Instructions:

1. Include all the ingredients in a pot with six cups of water.
2. Reduce the soup to three cups and consume one bowl per serving, three times a day.

How to consume:

Consume orally. Drink three cups a day until symptoms have improved.

Joint Pain

Joint pain can be caused by a number of reasons, including imbalanced diets and weakening of the bones.

Chinese Remedy:

Ingredients:

two Quails, cleaned

two spoons of Cooking wine,

60 grams of Job's tears

200 grams of papaya (cut into cubes)

15 grams of Acanthopanacis root barks

3 small cubes of ginger.

Instructions:

1. Start with eight cups of water and boil all the ingredients.
2. Reduce the soup to two cups.
3. Add a little salt and the wine.
4. Consume daily.

How to consume:

Orally, consume one cup a day for at least ten days.

Vomiting

Vomiting is characterized by the inability of the body to digest food and the body discards the food in the form of liquid through the mouth. Belching is a very common ailment and easily treatable.

Chinese Remedy:

Ingredients:

> 20 grams of dried ginger
> 20 grams of cinnamon bark
> 20 grams of garlic
> 200 grams of mutton; make sure you cut the mutton into small pieces.

Instructions:

1. Take the cinnamon stick and ginger, take four cups of water and boil these ingredients. Reduce to one cup. Keep aside.
2. In another pot prepare soup with mutton and crushed garlic.

3. Add in the herbal tea and simmer for ten minutes.

4. Serve one bowl daily.

How to consume:

Orally, consume one cup a day for at three days.

Ulcer

Ulcer is caused by the discontinuity in the bodily membrane that impedes the normal bodily functions of the body.

Chinese Remedy:

Ingredients:

80 grams of money head mushrooms

80 grams of deng shen

40 grams of dried red snail

3 honey dates

300 grams of lean pork

1 small piece of citrus peel (soaked in water for 15 minutes and cleaned)

Instructions:

1. Take ten cups of water in a pot and boil the ingredients until the water
2. Reduced two cups.
3. Add salt and serve.

How to consume:

Orally, consume one cup a day for at least ten days.

Headache

Cephalalgia, more commonly known as a headache, is characterized by pain in the head and the neck region. Headaches can also be a symptom for several other conditions, such as high blood pressure and insomnia.

Chinese Remedy:

Ingredients:

320 grams of spinach
200 grams of Chinese celery
80 grams of snow ear mushrooms
sesame oil to drizzle

Instructions:

1. Soak mushrooms in water until they soften a little bit.
2. Boil in five cups of water.
3. Add some salt and sesame oil before serving.

How to consume:

Orally, consume one to two cups a day when you have a headache.

Hypertension

Hypertension is also commonly known as high blood pressure. It is characterized by high pressure of blood flowing in the arteries.

Chinese Remedy:

Ingredients:

> one cucumber (cubed)
>
> 30 grams of seaweed
>
> one piece of firm tofu (drained and cubed)
>
> 120 grams of Chinese celery
>
> one spoon of dried shrimp and
>
> one teaspoon of grated garlic

Instructions:

1. Rinse all the ingredients. Soak and rinse the dried shrimp. Cut it into pieces.
2. Stir fry garlic and shrimp in oil for one minute.
3. Add tofu and brown.
4. Add the rest of the ingredients and plate.

How to consume:

Orally, consume one plate or more every day. No restriction.

Night Sweat

Sweating profusely in the night is common in men and women. Night sweat may be caused by a number of reasons, including infections, medication and cancer.

Chinese Remedy:

Ingredients:

>   15 grams of Wheat
>   9 grams of Astragalus
>   9 grams of Ophiopogonis Radix
>   honey for sweetness, if you want
>   around 20 red dates
>   60 grams of lack glutinous rice

Instructions:

1. Boil the ingredients in six cups of water and reduce the water to three cups.
2. Add honey for sweetness.
3. Strain and drink one cup daily.

How to consume:

Orally, consume one cup a day for at least ten days.

Menopausal Discomfort

Menopausal Discomfort is commonly experienced by females between 40 to 50 years of age as they reach their menopause. Symptoms include restlessness and burning in th heart.

Chinese Remedy:

Ingredients:

> 60 grams of lotus seeds
> 10 grams of licorice

Instructions:

1. Boil in two cups of water and reduce to one cup.
2. Strain and drink as tea, once a day.

How to consume:

Orally, consume one cup a day throughout your menstrual cycle.

Stomach Pain

Stomach pain may be caused by indigestion and fullness or belching. Often referred to as cramps, it is common and easily treatable.

Chinese Remedy:

Ingredients:

> 150 grams of lean pork (cut into small pieces)
>
> 320 grams of bok choy
>
> 12 grams of nutgrass
>
> 15 grams of white peony
>
> 11 grams of Chinese palm tree
>
> 8 grams of hare's ear

Instructions:

1. Take around twelve cups of water and boil the above ingredients until the soup reduces to two cups.
2. Add some salt and serve.

How to consume:

Orally, consume two cups a day. No restrictions, you can consume more if the symptoms don't improve.

Conclusion

Like you have read, Chinese medicine uses herbs to cure common ailments that not only offer health. It also promotes wellness and quick as well as long term cures to different ailments including blood pressure and stomach pains. Chinese herbal remedies use some commonly used ingredients to offer health. Mostly consisting of teas and soups, the recipes are easy to make.

Some of the recipes can be used on a daily basis without any restriction because these medicines are basically harmless. Decades of studies and testing of these medicines through centuries have perfected these medicines for the use of the public. Now, you can make these recipes at home without any help; just gather the ingredients and prepare a concoction that you can consume orally.

The beauty of the Chinese medicine is in the ease of its consumption; as you must have noticed, there is nothing more than orally consuming the liquid prepared for a prescribed number of days and you can restore your health. Since it has been used for centuries, the Chinese medicine has now, through a serial of trial and error, perfected.

If these medicines have been curing people for such a long time; isn't it time we gave up heavy allopathic medications and tried some herbal recipes that have proven to permanently cure illnesses for which even modern medicine still has no permanent cure?

www.ingramcontent.com/pod-product-compliance
Lightning Source LLC
Chambersburg PA
CBHW040312010626
45792CB00022B/242